Cenforce Usage For Men To Get The Most Out Of Sexual Health

Felix Eriksson

© 2024 Felix Eriksson. All rights reserved.

Disclaimer

The data gave on this stage is to instructive and educational purposes as it were. It isn't expected as a substitute for proficient clinical counsel, conclusion, or treatment. Continuously look for the counsel of your doctor or other qualified wellbeing supplier with any inquiries you might have in regards to an ailment. Never ignore proficient clinical guidance or postpone in looking for it in light of something you have perused on this stage.

Contents

Introduction 1

Uses 8

Side Effect 13

Interactions 17

Dosage 22

FAQ 26

Introduction

Cenforce is a medication designed to treat erectile dysfunction (ED) and impotence. Its active ingredient, Sildenafil, works by relaxing the muscles and blood vessels in the penis, enhancing blood flow and making it easier for men to achieve an erection.

Mechanism of Action

Sildenafil citrate, the key component of Cenforce, functions as a phosphodiesterase type 5 (PDE5) inhibitor. By blocking the PDE5 enzyme, it promotes the relaxation of smooth muscles and the dilation of blood vessels in the penis, which increases blood flow and facilitates an erection in response to sexual arousal.

Available Forms and Dosage

Cenforce is available in various strengths, including 25 mg, 50 mg, and 100 mg. The usual starting dose is typically 50 mg, but this can be adjusted based on individual response and tolerance. It is generally recommended to take the medication about 30 minutes to an hour before sexual activity.

Administration Guidelines

How to Take: Cenforce should be taken orally with water. It is advisable to avoid high-fat meals, as they can delay the medication's effectiveness.

Frequency: It is generally not recommended to take Cenforce more than once a day.

Potential Side Effects

Common side effects may include:

- Headache
- Flushing
- Indigestion
- Nasal congestion
- Dizziness
- Visual disturbances

In rare instances, serious side effects can occur, such as priapism (an erection lasting longer than 4 hours), severe changes in vision, or sudden hearing loss. If any of these serious side effects occur, immediate medical attention is necessary.

Precautions

Before using Cenforce, consider the following:

Health Conditions: Inform your healthcare provider about any existing health issues, particularly heart conditions, blood pressure irregularities, or liver and kidney disorders.

Drug Interactions: Cenforce may interact with certain medications, especially nitrates used for chest pain, which can lead to dangerously low blood pressure.

Alcohol and Grapefruit: Excessive alcohol consumption and grapefruit juice can impact the effectiveness and side effects of the medication.

Consultation

It is essential to consult a healthcare provider before starting Cenforce to ensure it is appropriate for you and to discuss any potential risks or interactions with other medications you may be taking.

What is Cenforce 200 mg?

Cenforce 200 mg is available in three strengths, all containing Sildenafil, which is similar to Viagra. The differences among these tablets are straightforward. The lighter variant, Cenforce 100 mg (the blue tablet), contains 100 mg of Sildenafil, the same amount found in Kamagra and Viagra. In contrast, the red Cenforce 150 mg and the black Cenforce 200 mg offer higher dosages. Cenforce pills are effective for approximately 4-6 hours and should be taken 30 minutes before sexual activity. The flavor of Cenforce is mild, and it is considered a neutral product. These pills are manufactured by Shree Venkatesh, the original creator of the formulation.

Why Choose Cenforce 200 mg?*

Cenforce 200 mg operates similarly to Viagra, sharing the same active ingredient, Sildenafil, along with Dapoxetine. Some users report that Cenforce is more effective than

Viagra, with fewer side effects compared to other erectile dysfunction medications. This has contributed to its popularity among men experiencing erection issues. Cenforce enhances sexual pleasure and ensures a firm erection is achieved and maintained. The active ingredient, Sildenafil, ensures the dilation of blood vessels, allowing for increased blood flow to the penis, resulting in quicker and easier erections. Importantly, Cenforce tablets have undergone thorough testing to ensure their safety.

Warning

Before taking Cenforce 200mg, it is important to consult your doctor or pharmacist, especially if you have a sensitivity to the medication or a history of allergies. The product may contain inactive ingredients that could trigger allergic reactions or other issues. For more information, please reach out to your pharmacist.

Administration of Cenforce 200mg

Always review the leaflet provided by your pharmacist before taking Cenforce 200mg with each refill. If you have any questions, do not hesitate to ask your doctor or pharmacist.

To treat erectile dysfunction, take Cenforce 200mg as prescribed by your physician. It is typically taken when needed, ideally 30 minutes to 4 hours before sexual activity, with 1 hour being the most effective timing. Do not exceed two doses in a 24-hour period.

Be aware that a high-fat meal may reduce the effectiveness of Cenforce 200mg. The appropriate dosage will depend on your medical conditions, your response to treatment, and any other medications you may be taking. Make sure to inform your doctor and pharmacist about all products you are using, including prescription medications, over-the-counter drugs, and herbal supplements.

Cenforce 200mg

Cenforce 100mg (Tadalafil TDA - Generic Cialis) is a leading product for enhancing erections!

Cenforce 200mg is manufactured in India by Centurion Laboratories, a well-known pharmaceutical company. This generic version contains 100mg of Tadalafil and has been available from the manufacturer since its release. Cenforce 200mg is a reliable option for those seeking effective treatment.

Cenforce 200mg tablets assist many men with erectile dysfunction by facilitating blood flow to the penis, which is essential for achieving an erection during sexual stimulation. When combined with sexual arousal, Cenforce 200mg promotes effective blood circulation, resulting in a strong and lasting erection. This is why it is widely regarded as a complete alternative to Cialis.

How Does Cenforce 200mg Work?

Cenforce 200mg tablets contain Tadalafil, the active ingredient that enhances blood flow to the penis, thereby improving erections. This powerful compound works by relaxing the smooth muscles in the blood vessels, allowing for increased blood flow into the cavernous bodies of the penis. As a result, users experience improved quality and duration of erections. Often referred to as a "weekend tablet," Cenforce 200mg is known for its long-lasting effects.

Uses

Cenforce, which contains sildenafil citrate, is primarily utilized for the following purposes:

Erectile Dysfunction (ED)

This is the primary indication for Cenforce. Erectile dysfunction is a condition where a man struggles to achieve or maintain an erection adequate for sexual intercourse. Cenforce aids in this by enhancing blood flow to the penis, enabling an erection in response to sexual arousal.

Mechanism: Cenforce promotes erection by amplifying the effects of nitric oxide, a substance that relaxes blood vessels in the penis.

Administration: It is generally taken 30-60 minutes prior to sexual activity, with effects lasting up to 4-6 hours, although this can vary.

Effectiveness: The medication is most effective when combined with sexual stimulation; it does not act as an aphrodisiac and does not enhance sexual desire.

Pulmonary Arterial Hypertension (PAH)

While not its primary application, sildenafil (the active component in Cenforce) is also prescribed under different brand names (such as Revatio) for the treatment of pulmonary arterial hypertension. PAH is characterized by elevated blood pressure in the lung arteries, which can result in shortness of breath and other symptoms. Sildenafil works by relaxing and widening the blood vessels in the lungs, thereby improving blood flow and reducing the heart's workload.

Mechanism: Sildenafil alleviates PAH symptoms by dilating lung blood vessels, lowering pressure in the pulmonary arteries, and easing the heart's pumping effort.

Usage: This condition is typically treated with a different formulation and dosage than that used for ED. Revatio is the brand name for PAH treatment, but its mechanism of action is similar to that of Cenforce.

Raynaud's Phenomenon

Sildenafil has been investigated in some studies for the treatment of Raynaud's phenomenon, a condition that restricts blood flow to extremities (such as fingers and toes), causing them to appear pale or blue. It may improve blood circulation in these areas, although it is not commonly prescribed for this purpose.

Mechanism: Sildenafil may enhance blood flow to the extremities affected by Raynaud's, but this application is less common and not standard practice.

Effectiveness: Ongoing research is being conducted, and this use is generally regarded as experimental or off-label.

Off-Label Uses

Cenforce may occasionally be prescribed off-label for other conditions related to blood flow or sexual health issues. However, these uses should be discussed with a healthcare provider to ensure safety and efficacy.

Consultation for Use

It is crucial to use Cenforce only under the supervision of a healthcare professional to confirm its suitability for your specific condition and to avoid potential interactions or side effects.

Additional Considerations

Sexual Health: In addition to addressing erectile dysfunction (ED), enhancing sexual performance can positively influence psychological well-being and relationship satisfaction.

Lifestyle Factors: To achieve optimal results, it is essential to consider lifestyle changes such as reducing alcohol consumption, quitting smoking, and managing stress alongside medication.

Precautions and Contraindications

Cardiovascular Health: Men with heart conditions or those taking certain medications (such as nitrates) should exercise caution, as combining these can result in significant drops in blood pressure.

Kidney and Liver Function: Individuals with liver or kidney issues may need dosage adjustments and careful monitoring.

Other Medications: Be sure to inform your healthcare provider about all medications you are currently taking, including over-the-counter drugs and supplements.

Potential Side Effects

Common: Possible side effects include headaches, flushing, nasal congestion, and digestive problems.

Serious: Although rare, serious side effects can occur, such as prolonged erections (priapism), sudden changes in vision, or hearing loss. These conditions require immediate medical attention.

If you have specific concerns or medical conditions, it is advisable to consult your healthcare provider to determine whether Cenforce is appropriate and safe for you.

Side Effect

Here's a detailed breakdown of the side effects associated with Cenforce:

Common Side Effects

These effects are generally mild and temporary:

Headache: Often caused by the widening of blood vessels.

Flushing: A sensation of warmth or redness in the face, neck, or chest.

Indigestion: Mild stomach upset or heartburn.

Nasal Congestion: A stuffy or runny nose.

Dizziness: Feelings of light-headedness or unsteadiness, especially when standing up quickly.

Visual Disturbances: Temporary changes in vision, such as a bluish tint or increased sensitivity to light.

Less Common Side Effects

These effects are less frequent but may occur:

Muscle or Back Pain: Discomfort or aching in the muscles or back.

Rash: Skin irritation or itching.

Sleep Issues: Difficulty falling asleep or staying asleep.

Serious Side Effects

These are rare but require immediate medical attention:

Priapism: A painful erection lasting more than 4 hours, which necessitates urgent medical treatment to prevent long-term damage.

Sudden Vision Loss: Partial or complete loss of vision in one or both eyes, potentially indicating a serious condition like non-arteritic anterior ischemic optic neuropathy (NAION).

Sudden Hearing Loss: A rapid decrease or loss of hearing, possibly accompanied by ringing in the ears (tinnitus).

Chest Pain or Severe Dizziness: These symptoms may signal cardiovascular issues and require prompt evaluation.

Managing Side Effects

For Minor Effects: Staying hydrated, avoiding alcohol, and taking the medication with food (if recommended) may help alleviate common side effects.

For Serious Effects: Seek immediate medical assistance if you experience severe symptoms such as priapism, sudden vision or hearing loss, or chest pain.

Precautions

Health Conditions: Inform your healthcare provider about any pre-existing health conditions, especially cardiovascular issues, kidney, or liver disorders.

Drug Interactions: Be aware of potential interactions with other medications, particularly nitrates, which can lead to a dangerous drop in blood pressure.

Lifestyle Considerations: Limit excessive alcohol consumption and grapefruit juice, as they can affect the effectiveness and side effect profile of Cenforce.

If you have any concerns about side effects or if they persist or worsen, it's essential to contact a healthcare professional for guidance and support.

Interactions

Cenforce, which contains sildenafil citrate, can interact with various substances, potentially affecting its effectiveness or increasing the risk of side effects. Below is a comprehensive overview of possible interactions:

Nitrates

Examples: Nitroglycerin, isosorbide dinitrate, isosorbide mononitrate.

Effect: Using Cenforce alongside nitrates can cause a significant drop in blood pressure, leading to dizziness, fainting, or even a heart attack.

Advice: Avoid taking Cenforce if you are currently using nitrates or have been prescribed them for chest pain.

Alpha-Blockers

Examples: Doxazosin, prazosin, terazosin.

Effect: These medications, often prescribed for high blood pressure or benign prostatic hyperplasia (BPH), can also lower blood pressure. When taken with Cenforce, the risk of hypotension (low blood pressure) increases.

Advice: If you are on alpha-blockers, your doctor may need to adjust the dosage of either medication or monitor your blood pressure closely.

Other Blood Pressure Medications

Examples: Certain antihypertensives, including some diuretics and beta-blockers.

Effect: These medications can also lower blood pressure, and combining them with Cenforce may enhance this effect.

Advice: Regular blood pressure monitoring is advisable if you are taking other medications that lower blood pressure.

HIV Protease Inhibitors

Examples: Ritonavir, saquinavir.

Effect: These drugs can elevate sildenafil levels in the bloodstream, potentially intensifying the effects and side effects of Cenforce.

Advice: Dosage adjustments may be required, and your healthcare provider will monitor you for increased side effects.

Antifungal Medications

   - **Examples:** Ketoconazole, itraconazole.

   - **Effect:** These can also raise sildenafil levels, increasing the likelihood of side effects.

   - **Advice:** Your healthcare provider may need to modify your Cenforce dosage or monitor you closely for side effects.

6. **Antibiotics**

   - **Examples:** Erythromycin, clarithromycin.

Effect: Certain antibiotics can increase sildenafil levels, altering its side effect profile.

Advice: Inform your doctor if you are taking these antibiotics so they can adjust the dosage if necessary.

Grapefruit Juice

Effect: Grapefruit juice can inhibit liver enzymes that metabolize sildenafil, raising its concentration in the blood and potentially increasing side effects.

Advice: Avoid consuming grapefruit juice while taking Cenforce.

Alcohol

Effect: Alcohol can amplify the blood-pressure-lowering effects of Cenforce, increasing the risk of dizziness and fainting. It may also hinder your ability to achieve an erection.

Advice: Limit alcohol intake while using Cenforce.

General Recommendations

Inform Your Doctor: Always disclose all medications (including over-the-counter drugs and supplements) you are taking to your healthcare provider before starting Cenforce.

Monitor for Side Effects: Be alert for any unusual symptoms or side effects, especially when initiating or adjusting medication dosages.

Consult Your Healthcare Provider: If you have questions about drug interactions or are considering new medications or supplements, seek personalized advice from your healthcare provider.

Dosage

Cenforce, which contains sildenafil citrate, is available in multiple dosages to accommodate varying patient needs and responses. Here's a summary of the standard dosages:

Cenforce 25 mg

Indication: Often suggested as an initial dose, especially for individuals who may be more sensitive to the medication or for older patients.

Administration: Usually taken 30-60 minutes before engaging in sexual activity.

Effectiveness: Can be modified based on personal tolerance and response.

Cenforce 50 mg

Indication: Frequently prescribed as a starting dose for most men, providing a balance between efficacy and tolerability.

Administration: Taken orally approximately 30-60 minutes prior to sexual activity.

Effectiveness: Adjustments can be made based on individual response.

Cenforce 100 mg

Indication: Typically recommended for those who do not achieve satisfactory results with lower doses, offering a higher dose of sildenafil for enhanced effectiveness.

Administration: Taken 30-60 minutes before sexual activity.

Effectiveness: Higher doses may increase the likelihood of side effects, so medical supervision is advised.

Cenforce 150 mg

Indication: Generally used when lower doses are ineffective; not usually the first option due to a greater risk of side effects.

Administration: Taken at the same timing as other doses, prior to sexual activity.

Effectiveness: The increased risk of side effects requires close monitoring by a healthcare professional.

Cenforce 200 mg

Indication: The highest standard dose, reserved for situations where other dosages have not been effective. This dose is typically used when the benefits outweigh the potential risks.

Administration: Taken 30-60 minutes before sexual activity.

Effectiveness: Higher risk of side effects necessitates cautious use.

Dosage Guidelines

Start Low: It is generally recommended to begin with a lower dose (25 mg or 50 mg) and adjust based on effectiveness and tolerability.

Frequency: Cenforce is usually taken once daily, with timing tailored to individual needs and medical advice.

Adjustments: Any changes in dosage should be made under the supervision of a healthcare provider to avoid adverse effects.

Consult Your Healthcare Provider

Individual Needs: The appropriate dosage may differ based on personal health conditions, other medications, and treatment response.

Medical Advice: Always follow your healthcare provider's recommendations regarding dosage to ensure safety and effectiveness.

If you have any questions or concerns about your dosage or how Cenforce may affect you, please reach out to your healthcare provider for personalized advice and guidance.

FAQ

Frequently Asked Questions (FAQ) about Cenforce**

What is Cenforce used for?

Cenforce is mainly prescribed for the treatment of erectile dysfunction (ED) in men. It aids in achieving and sustaining an erection by enhancing blood flow to the penis. In some instances, it may also be used to manage pulmonary arterial hypertension (PAH), although this typically involves a different formulation and dosage.

How should Cenforce be taken?

Cenforce is taken orally, usually in tablet form with water. It is generally advised to take it approximately 30-60 minutes before sexual activity. The effects can last for about 4-6 hours. It is important not to exceed one dose per day.

What should I do if I miss a dose?

Cenforce is typically taken on an as-needed basis, so missing a dose is not usually a significant issue. If you are on a regular dosing schedule and miss a dose, take it as soon as you remember. However, if it's nearly time for your next dose, skip the missed one and do not take two doses at once.

What are the common side effects of Cenforce?

Common side effects may include headaches, flushing, indigestion, nasal congestion, dizziness, and visual disturbances. These effects are generally mild and temporary.

What serious side effects should I be aware of?

Serious side effects that require immediate medical attention include priapism (an erection lasting longer than 4 hours), sudden loss of vision or hearing, and severe chest pain.

www.ingramcontent.com/pod-product-compliance
Lightning Source LLC
Chambersburg PA
CBHW070958220526
45471CB00007B/3082